Yoga Practice

In Fitness

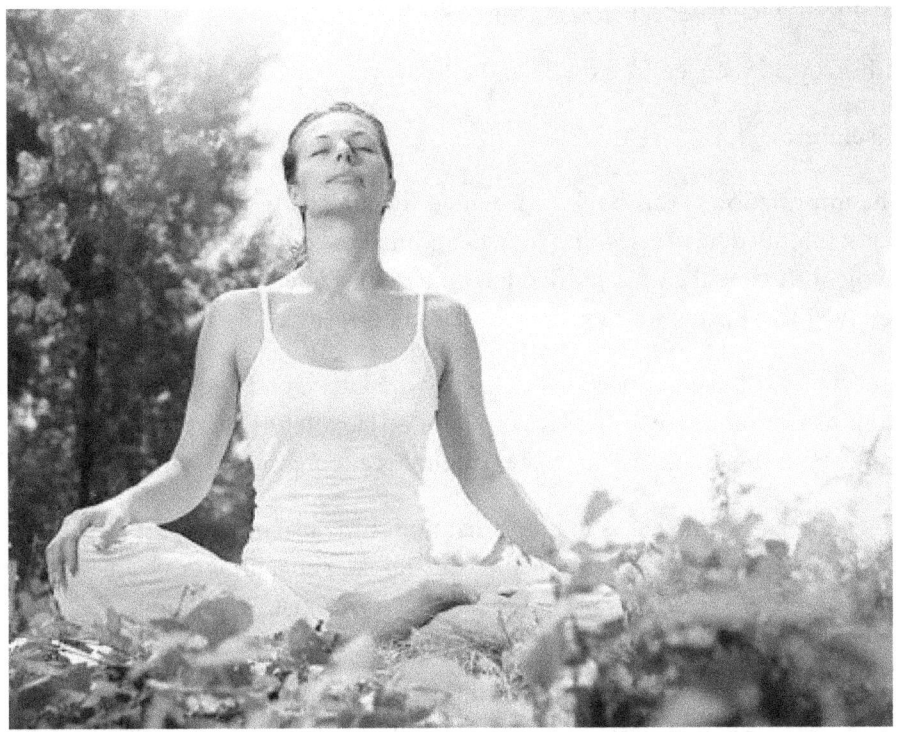

Health Learning Series

M. Usman

Mendon Cottage Books

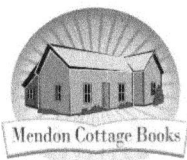

JD-Biz Publishing

Disclaimer

The information is this book is provided for informational purposes only. It is not intended to be used and medical advice or a substitute for proper medical treatment by a qualified health care provider. The information is believed to be accurate as presented based on research by the author.

The contents have not been evaluated by the U.S. Food and Drug Administration or any other Government or Health Organization and the contents in this book are not to be used to treat cure or prevent disease.

The author or publisher is not responsible for the use or safety of any diet, procedure or treatment mentioned in this book. The author or publisher is not responsible for errors or omissions that may exist.

Warning

The Book is for informational purposes only and before taking on any diet, treatment or medical procedure, it is recommended to consult with your primary health care provider.

Our books are available at

1. Amazon.com
2. Barnes and Noble
3. Itunes
4. Kobo
5. Smashwords
6. Google Play Books

Table of Contents

Preface

Most of us are habituated to seeking outside of ourselves for nirvana. Today, we live in a world that makes us believe that outer accomplishments and attainments can give us what we want. Yet, every now and then our experiences illustrate that nothing external can entirely satisfy the unfathomable yearning within, for more. Regardless of the time, nevertheless, we discover ourselves endeavoring toward that which always seems to lie just outside our reach. We are always focusing on *doing* rather than *being*, in action rather than sentience and awareness. It is difficult for us to imagine a state of far-reaching serenity and tranquility in which thoughts and feelings cease to dance in eternal motion. There is no blinking the fact, that through such a state of peacefulness, we can trace a level of happiness and understanding difficult to attain otherwise.

Yoga is a simple course of reversing the usual outward flow of energy and realization. This is so the mind develops a vibrant center of direct insight, which is no longer reliant on the imperfect senses, but proficient enough to actually experience the Truth.

The next sections discuss yoga, its goals, benefits, and plans in detail.

Getting Started

Chapter # 1: Introduction

Yoga is a physical, psychological, and spiritual practice or discipline. It can be regarded as an ascetic discipline where a portion of which, including breath control, simple contemplation, and the practice of definite bodily stances, is extensively practiced for fitness and relaxation.

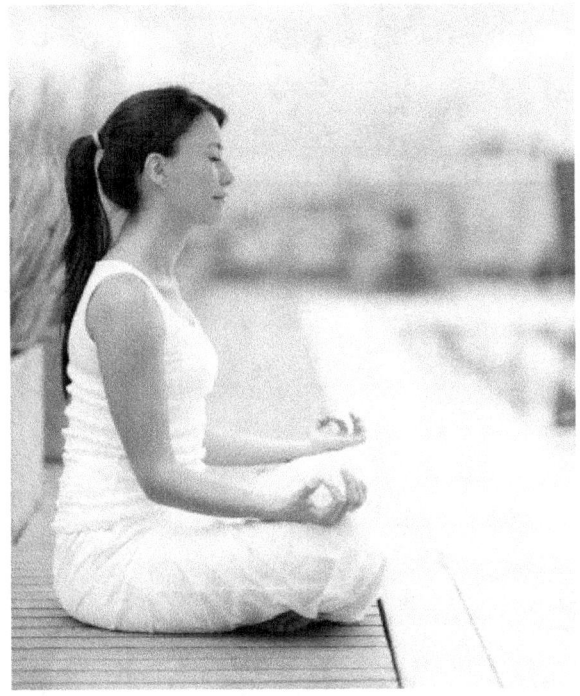

By performing the step-by-step methods of Yoga and also through blind faith, we come to discern our coherence with the Infinite Intelligence, Supremacy, and Bliss which gives life to all and which is the essence of our own Self. In the past epochs, numerous advanced practices of Yoga were little understood or practiced due to mankind's inadequate familiarity with the forces that run the universe. Today, scientific study is speedily altering the way we see all God's creatures and ourselves. The outdated money-oriented notion of life has disappeared with the discovery that matter and energy are fundamentally one. Every existing element can be concentrated to an arrangement or form of energy, which intermingles and interrelates with other forms. Some of today's most renowned physicists go a step further ascertaining mindfulness and consciousness as the essential ground of all being. Thus, modern science is approving the antique values and philosophies of Yoga, which declare that unity pervades the universe.

Chapter # 2: Goals

The definitive goal of Yoga is moksha (deliverance and emancipation), though the precise definition depends on the theoretical or spiritual system with which it is conjugated.

Yoga has five basic meanings:

- Yoga as a methodical technique for achieving an objective

- Yoga as practices of monitoring the body and the thoughts

- Yoga as an appellation of one of the systems of viewpoint (darśana)

- Yoga in assembly with other words, similar to hatha, mantra etc. symbolizing to societies, specifying in particular, the skills of yoga

- Yoga as the goal of Yoga practice

Agreeing to David Gordon White from the 5th century CE onwards, the central doctrines of "yoga" were more or less in place, and disparities of these principles established in various forms over the years.

Yoga as a scrutiny of discernment and understanding, as the intensification and development of mindfulness, as a pathway to sagacity and omniscience, as a procedure for entering into other bodies, producing multiple bodies, and the accomplishment of other supernatural accomplishments, have all been discussed in various Hindu religious books.

Chapter # 3: Paths of Yoga

The word yoga itself means "union": of the distinct realization or soul with the Universal Consciousness or Spirit. Although several people consider yoga only as bodily exercises — the asanas or postures that have extended widespread fame in modern times — these are essentially the shallowest characteristic of this philosophical science of describing the immeasurable abilities of the human mind and soul.

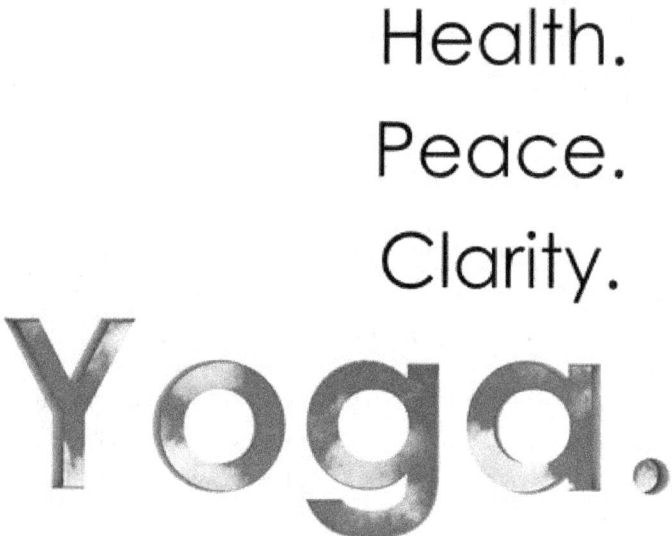

There are numerous paths of Yoga that hint toward this objective with each one a dedicated division of one wide-ranging system:

1.   Hatha Yoga — a scheme of physical postures, or asanas, whose greater purpose is to cleanse the body, giving one awareness and control over its internal states and rendering it fit for meditation.

2.　　Karma Yoga — self-sacrificing amenity to others as part of one's larger Self, without attachment to the consequences; and the enactment of all movements with the realization of God as the Doer.

3.　　Mantra Yoga — concentrating the mindfulness within through japa or the recurrence of definite universal root-word sounds on behalf of a particular aspect of Spirit.

4.　　Bhakti Yoga — all-surrendering dedication through which one endeavors to understand and love the spirituality in every single being and in the whole lot, thus upholding an interminable worship.

5.　　Jnana (Gyana) Yoga — the pathway of astuteness and understanding, which gives emphasis to the solicitation of discriminative astuteness and intellect, to accomplish spiritual emancipation.

6.　　Raja Yoga — the majestic or uppermost pathway of Yoga, which conglomerates the spirit of all the other pathways.

At the core of the Raja Yoga structure, harmonizing and amalgamating these various methods is the practice of fixed, scientific approaches of meditation that allow one to recognize, from the very commencement of one's hard work, previews of the final goal — cognizant union with the inexhaustibly delightful Spirit.

The fastest and most operational method to the goal of Yoga employs those procedures of contemplation that deal unswervingly with vigor and awareness. It is this shortest method that exemplifies Kriya Yoga, the specific form of Raja Yoga contemplation, taught by Paramahansa Yogananda.

Chapter # 4: Benefits of Yoga

Developed in India thousands of eons ago, yoga has developed into an all the time more popular form of workout in the United States. Whether yoga's recent upsurge in admiration stems from a rise in stress levels or the following of a Hollywood fashion, yoga supplies much assistance to those who integrate it into their daily lives.

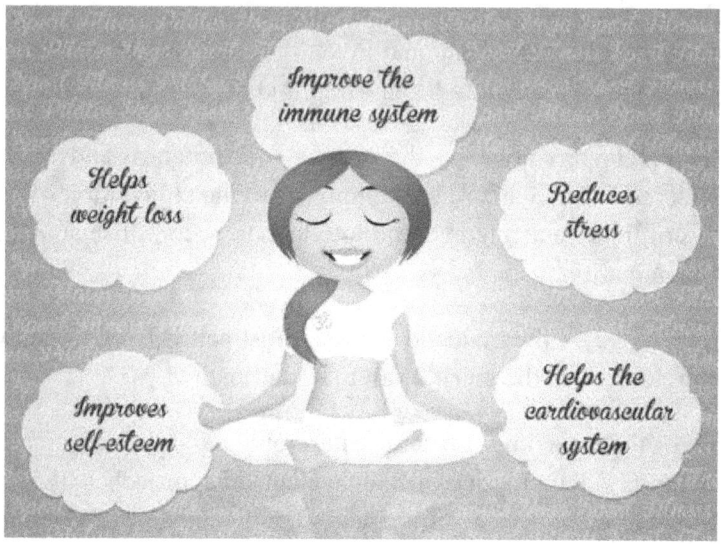

"Yoga is a remedial system of concept and practice. The objective of yoga is to produce strength, cognizance and synchronization in both the mind and physique," explains Natalie Nevins, D.O., a board-certified osteopathic family physician and certified Kundalini Yoga instructor in Hollywood, California. "As an osteopathic doctor, I stress a lot of my dynamisms on defensive medicine and practices, and in the body's ability to reconcile itself. Yoga is a great means for staying vigorous since it is based on analogous philosophies."

Though there are more than one hundred diverse kinds, or schools, of yoga, most assemblies are typically comprised of breathing calisthenics, exercises, contemplation, and presumptuous postures (sometimes called asana or poses) that expanse and stretch numerous muscle groups.

In the words of Dr. Nevins, the moderation procedures amalgamated in yoga can decrease chronic pain, such as lower back pain, inflammation, annoyances, and carpal tunnel syndrome. Yoga can also lead to lower blood pressure and diminish insomnia.

Agreeing with Dr. Nevins, other physical benefits of yoga include:

- Amplified flexibility

- Improved muscle strength and tone

- Improved respiration, vigor, and liveliness

- The conservation of a well-adjusted metabolic rate

- Weight reduction

- Cardio and cardiovascular health

- Value-added athletic enactment

- Fortification from injury

Apart from the collection of physical remunerations, one of the best benefits of yoga is how it helps an individual cope with stress, which has been identified to have demoralizing effects on the body and mind. Stress can divulge itself in many ways, together with back or neck pain, slumbering problems, annoyances, drug abuse, and an inability to quintessence. Yoga can be very operative in increasing coping expertise and accomplishment of a more positive outlook on life.

Contradictory to more old-style forms of exercise, yoga's amalgamation of contemplation and breathing helps a person improve and increase his/her psychological well-being. Consistent yoga practice creates psychological clarity and tranquility, increases body consciousness, dismisses chronic stress configurations, relaxes the mind, centers thoughtfulness, and improves attentiveness. Body and self-awareness, in particular, are very advantageous for the reason that it can help with early discovery of bodily complications or illnesses and allow for early precautionary action.

For the reason that there are so many different kinds of yoga practices, it is likely for anyone to start. Whether you're a couch potato or a specialized athlete, size and appropriateness levels do not matter for the reason that there are amendments for every yoga pose; a learner class in every style. The notion is to reconnoiter your limits, not strive for some pretzel-like perfection.

Yoga can be adept to progress overall interests, to develop equipoise, to put to rights and avert wounds, to make sturdier muscles and to open the body for contemplation. It is a prodigious way to get in tune with your body and your inner self. Yoga's increasing attractiveness is evidence that many people rate an exercise system that occupies the mind, body, and spirit in equal measure. If you've under no circumstances done yoga beforehand, give it a shot and perceive what it can sort out for you.

Physiological Benefits of Yoga:

The physiological benefits of yoga can be classified as under:

1. Steady autonomic nervous system balance

2. Pulse rate diminutions

3. Respiratory rate reductions

4. Blood Pressure declines (of special importance for hypo reactors)

5. Galvanic Skin Response (GSR) intensifications

6. EEG - alpha waves increase (theta, delta, and beta waves also increase during various stages of meditation)

7. EMG activity reductions

8. Cardiovascular competence upsurges

9. Respiratory effectiveness increases

10. Gastrointestinal utility normalizes

11. Endocrine function normalizes

12. Excretory functions increases

13. Musculoskeletal elasticity and joint range of motion proliferation

14. Breath-holding time increases

15. Joint range of motion upsurge

16. Grip strength increases

17. Eye-hand synchronization improves

18. Legerdemain skills improve

19. Reaction time escalations

20. Posture improves

Psychological Benefits of Yoga

The psychological benefits of yoga can be classified as follows:

1. Somatic and kinesthetic responsiveness increase

2. Temper improves and idiosyncratic well-being increases

3. Self-acceptance and self-actualization increase

4. Social regulation increases

5. Nervousness and Downheartedness decreases

6. Aggression decreases

7. Attentiveness improves

8. Reminiscence improves

9. Thoughtfulness improves

10. Wisdom adeptness improves

11. Temperament improves

12. Communal services increases

13. Well-being increases

14. Somatic and kinesthetic cognizance increase

15. Responsiveness improves

16. Concentration improves

17. Retention improves

18. Book learning efficiency improves

7 Day Schedule

The 7 Day Yoga schedule is the most operative yoga aptness transformer on the market. Now, this is no ordinary schedule. You're going to focus, stream, and find out how and why you've been staying stuck in some disrupting patterns. This technique is going to help you out, and put you into a position of strength, inside and out, in just one week—30 minutes a day.

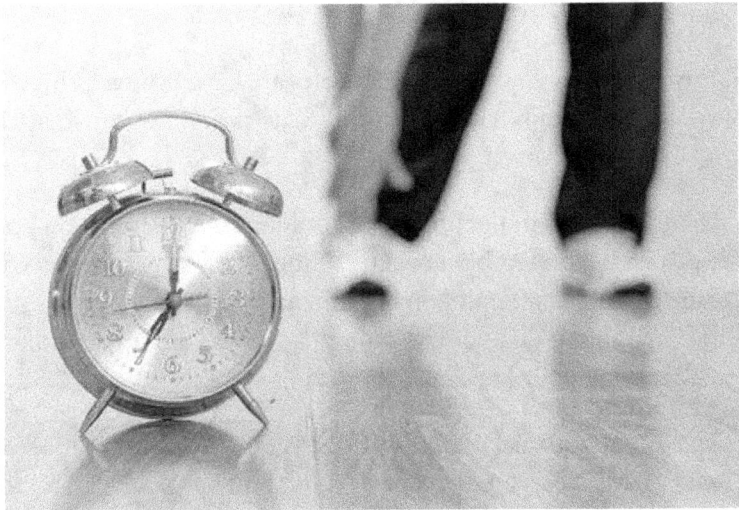

Equipment required:

- A yoga mat or non-slip surface

- Comfortable but form-fitting clothing

- Two 5-pound hand weights or soup cans

- A sturdy chair you can step up onto

Chapter # 1: Day 1

Learning configuration and alignment for arm balances aids you in finding alignment in every forte posture including revitalizations, and decreases the chances of injuries. Follow the simple instructions given below:

1. Begin with yogi squat. Pull your feet together beneath your body, heels should be touching, hands inflexibly planted on the ground at shoulder width distance away from each other.

2. Now rise on to your tread softly, elevating your hips as high as possible in the air. This elevation in the posture is key in attainment of lift in your poise.

3. Bring the knees to the uppermost point you can stretch on your upper limbs, preferably around the top side of the triceps. Now place the knees partially on the arm and partially sideways to the arm, imagining that you are clutching in on your arms, rather than just relaxing your knees there.

4. Gaze in the forward direction, around six inches in front of your hands. This aids you in keeping your shoulder blades lifted, which is crucial if you want to avoid falling on your face.

5. Swing your energy frontward till one foot rises off the floor. If this is as extreme as you can go, halt here for a small number of breaths, then put the first foot on the ground again and try again with the second foot.

6. If you sense equilibrium, carry on fluctuating to lift the second foot off the floor.

7. With both of your feet in the air, carry on gazing forward, clutching in on your arms with your thighs, and possibly trying to dash your feet together.

8. Clench for about five to twenty inhalations.

Chapter # 2: Day 2

Invigorate your body with a succession of sun salutations, and follow the simple steps given below:

1.   Start by standing on your your feet with legs relaxed, and then spread your toes. Make certain that your soles are fixed and stiffen your legs. Then, move your shoulders posterior and down and then you have to lift your ribcage.

2.   Breathe in through your nose and elevate your arms sideways, until your palms are in front of you. Spread out your arms overhead with your hands in supplication posture.

3.   Swan plunge to advancing bend; be certain to bend your knees particularly if you have constricted cramps. This will shield the back. Breathe out through your nose. Now open your upper limbs widely and bow at your diaphragm to a vertical forward curvature. Your hands should dash the ground if you can and in case this seems difficult, touch the front of your ankles.

4.   Breathe in through your nose and then move your hands next to your feet on the ground and place one foot back into a swipe. Keep the forward-facing knee straight over the ankle and keep the hind leg steady. Breathe out and carry the other foot backwards to form the downward-facing dog posture.

5.   Extend your fingers and apply force through your palms on the carpet, the width should be one shoulder apart. Lift your hips up in the direction of the ceiling, broadening your spine. Mildly flatten your legs, pushing your heels downwards into your mat as far as you can go.

6.   Breathe in and take your shoulders in a forward direction, unswervingly over your wrists, ranging well with your arms to formulate board position. Retain your thighs, robust and stable, and your feet should be bent and your abdomen drawn in.

7.   Breathe in and take your shoulder blades in a forward position straight over your wrists, spreading with your arms to formulate board position. Cling to your thighs, your feet bent and your abdomen drawn in.

8.   Breathe in and elevate your higher body to the cobra posture. Troll your shoulder blades backwards and spread the shoulder blades downwards and then press them in the direction of the ribcage. Your ribcage should be elevated and uncluttered and jostles should stay near to the physique. Make sure that your kneecaps are lifted and also secure your thighs. Your limbs and feet should be extended well.

9.   Breathe out and fold in your toes while twisting your knees and pushing back to a child's position. If probable, in the similar breath change your position directly back to downward-facing dog. Tug the abdomen up and near the hind of the spine.

10.   Now this is the point where we recap and repeat in opposite the first three positions that start the sun salutation.

11.   Now repeat the Sun Salutation on the other leg too.

Chapter # 3: Day 3, 4 & 5

Day 3

The Breath:

The breath is a very significant part of this structure. The movement from one posture to the next is always done in aggregation, either breathing in or breathing out on the movement. You can control the stride of the sequence by changing the number of breaths in each pose; just make sure to always move to the next pose on the accurate breath.

Upper body strength:

Start with the easiest overturn, tripod headstand. Follow the simple steps:

Place your skull and hands on the mat, uncurl your legs, and gait them, as near as you can, in the direction of your head. This is well thought-out as an overturn even though your feet are not in the air. If you feel prepared, repose your knees on your triceps, approaching again into tripod balance. From this point, you can toil on lifting one leg at an interval into the air.

Day 4

For stability and inner core strength:

1.   Squeeze together the internal thighs

2.   Involve the crosswise abdominisa

3.   Contract the hip flexors and the rectus abdominisa

By instantaneously engaging your internal muscles of your thighs, abdominals, and hip flexors, you will cultivate superior core métier, construct better steadiness, and strengthen a sensation of association all over your body.

Day 5

The following is a great workout and it will aid in tightening your muscles.

1. First you will need a yoga mat to lie on. A towel could serve the purpose.

2. Lie sideways on the yoga mat.

3. Twist your top knee backwards and make certain that it is in contour with your body.

4. Uncurl the front leg and elevate it out to some extent to the visible.

5. This will be the starting position.

6. Lift your hind limb until you reach a balanced state.

7. Hold your leg in this position for around 1 second.

8. Repeat the steps.

9. Change legs.

Chapter # 4: Day 6 & 7

Day 6:

This exercise will help you feel compassion for yourself; all you have to do is follow the simple steps:

1.   Hold your breath for about 5 to 10 minutes in a position where you are in a hanging state over your hind limbs and holding your elbows too.

2.   Now keeping your knee bent at a right angle, breathe in and out deeply for about 5 minutes while bending on your abdomen and then change legs.

3.   Now form the boat pose. You can also bend your knees during this step while trying to engage your core.

4.   Lie down flat on the floor and extend your arms in the air. Breathe in and out slowly.

5.   Place your forearms to the ground. Try to lift your body up and down keeping your head above the ground level.

Day 7:

In 60 powerful minutes practice, take your time to invigorate all portions of the body from end to end standing positions, balancing poses, abdominal movements and rotations. These postures will shape and build strength and flexibility as well as open your shoulders so the limb balance will be like the cherry on top as an outcome. Deeper hip work is extra dominant in this arrangement as we move to the last arm poise.

Doing yoga with the help of above mentioned equipment will help you learn the 7 Secrets to Yoga Body Success, instructions, tools and actions to take to ensure that you're clean, slender, fighting disease—and rocking your little black dress (or suit, guys) too!

Yoga is not all about weight loss. There comes a point when you drop too much weight and look and feel bad. Nevertheless, if you have additional weight to lose, this sequence will get you going, speedily. If you want to preserve a hale and hearty weight, ditto—this will serve the purpose.

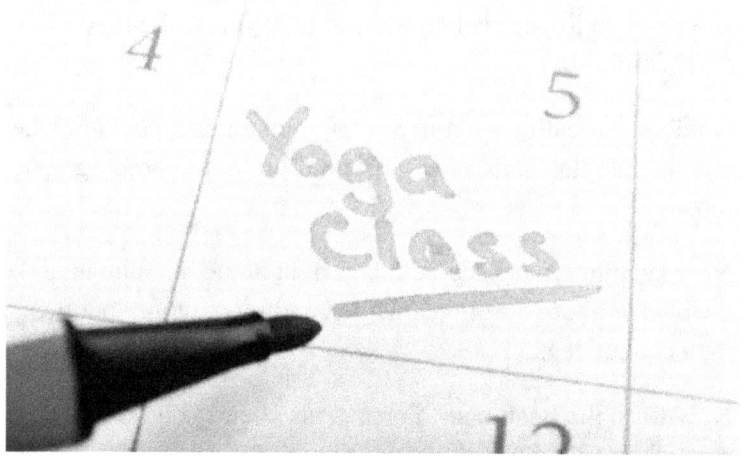

Given a time of 7 days, and the scheme, kick-start your fitness to a whole new level. You're about to go robust, and faster into your fitness, tendency, and detox than usual, which is good. At the end of the week, you will be nothing less than fit and fierce.

30 days Schedule

Chapter # 1: Week 1

Day 1: Daily Stretch Routine

Some days, it's just not probable to put in a full hour and a half of yoga. But most days will allow for this 10- to 15-minute arrangement that expanses the backbone, constrains, and hips, which are problematic areas for several people. Over time, you will see the optimistic and constructive effect these stretches have on your longer practice sessions. The first few pelvic slants expose any dashes of squat back pain, but after about 10 to 20 rounds, the aching is absent. Do the pelvic tilts gradually and keep going until the association feels fluid and good.

Day 2: Daily Stretch Routine + 3x Sun Salutations + Seated Stretches

Daily stretch routine:

Follow the daily stretch routine as described above.

Sun Salutations:

Sun salutations are a significant part of any flow style yoga practice. You may not even comprehend you are doing them, but many instructors use them as a warm up at the commencement of class or even base whole classes around them. If you learn this arrangement and sequence, it will really comfort you if you ever want to practice at home. One of the biggest difficulties to doing yoga on your own is reckoning what to do when you first get on your mat.

The Breath:

The breath is a very significant part of this structure. The movement from one posture to the next is always done in aggregation with either an inhale or an exhale. You can control the stride of the sequence by changing the number of breaths in each pose; just make sure to always move to the next pose on the accurate breath.

First Poses in the Sequence:

To inaugurate, bring yourself to the front edge of your mat in mountain pose - tadasana with the hands in Anjali mudra at your heart. This is conventionally where you might halt and set an intention for your drill if you chose to.

Breathe in - Bring the arms out to the sides and join your palms above your head in raised arms pose. Raise your stare to your hands and slide your shoulders away from your ears.

Seated stretches:

1. Start this sequence seated in Cobbler's Pose - Buddha Kona Sana.

2. Sit up on a blanket or block, whichever is more comfortable.

3. Come into a forward bend if possible.

Day 3: Daily Stretch Routine

Daily stretch routine:

Follow the daily stretch routine as described above.

Day 4: Daily Stretch Routine + 3x Sun Salutations + Standing Poses

Daily stretch routine:

Follow the daily stretch routine as described above.

Sun Salutations:

The procedure for sun salutations has already been discussed above.

Standing poses:

Try to bend your knees, coming up onto the balls of your feet, carrying the belly to rest on the thighs and the sit bones up high. Then descend your heels, uncurling the legs keeping the high upward rotation of the sit bones.

Also try twisting the arms slightly outwards to the side, moving the ribcage towards the thighs. Then you can straighten the arms.

Day 5: Daily Stretch Routine

Daily stretch routine:

Follow the daily stretch routine as described above.

Day 6: Daily Stretch Routine + 3x Sun Salutations + Standing Poses + Seated Stretches

Daily stretch routine:

Follow the daily stretch routine as described above.

Sun Salutations:

The procedure for sun salutations has already been discussed above.

Standing poses:

The procedure for standing poses has already been discussed above.

Seated stretches:

The procedure has been given in the previous chapter.

Day 7: Daily Stretch Routine:

Follow the daily stretch routine as described above.

Chapter # 2: Week 2

Day 1: Daily Stretch Routine:

The procedure has been given in the previous chapter.

Day 2: Daily Stretch Routine + 3x Moon Salutations + Standing Poses + Seated Stretches:

Initiate the arrangement standing in Mountain Pose – Tadasana.

Inhale - Hook the thumbs of your stretched out arms as you raise them up over the head. This variation of Raised Arms Pose -Urdhva Hastasana is a backbend, so try to grasp the arms toward the partition behind you.

Day 3: Daily Stretch Routine:

Follow the daily stretch routine as described above.

Day 4: Daily Stretch Routine + 3x Moon Salutations + Standing Poses + Standing Balances:

Daily stretch routine:

Follow the daily stretch routine as described above.

Moon Salutations:

The procedure for moon salutations has already been discussed above.

Standing poses:

The procedure for standing poses has already been discussed above.

Standing balances:

The important advantage of standing balances is that it strengthens the thighs (which have some practical uses).

Instructions:

1. From Mountain Pose – Tadasana bend the knees until the thighs are almost parallel to the floor.

2. Keep the butt low.

3. Bring the arms up towards the ceiling.

4. Bring a slight back bend into the upper back.

5. Hold 5-10 breaths

Day 5: Daily Stretch Routine:

Follow the daily stretch routine as described above.

Day 6: Daily Stretch Routine + 3x Moon Salutations + Standing Poses + Yoga for Abs:

Daily stretch routine:

Follow the daily stretch routine as described above.

Moon Salutations:

The procedure for moon salutations has already been discussed above.

Standing poses:

The procedure for standing poses has already been discussed above.

Yoga for Abs:

This categorization is made up of postures that will increase your core strength and help compress your abs. While doing yoga is not the finest way to get a six-pack, you can presume it will tone and make your stomach stronger. Solidification of your core can also help discharge back pain and mend your posture (nothing makes your belly look bigger than drooping!). Many of the postures recommended below are equilibriums, which are a great way to work the essential.

Let's get in full swing by coming onto all fours with your knees underneath your hips and your wrists underneath your shoulders. Do a few Cats-Cow Stretches to warm up, by bending your back on your inhalations and rounding your spine on your exhalations. Remember to keep your belly tight throughout both motions.

Day 7: Daily Stretch Routine:

Follow the daily stretch routine as described above.

Chapter # 3: Week 3

Follow the instructions for week 2 during this week.

Day 1: Daily Stretch Routine:

The procedure has been given in the previous chapter.

Day 2: Daily Stretch Routine + 3x Moon Salutations + Standing Poses + Seated Stretches:

Initiate the arrangement standing in Mountain Pose – Tadasana.

Inhale - Hook the thumbs of your stretched out arms as you raise them up over the head. This variation of Raised Arms Pose -Urdhva Hastasana is a backbend, so try to grasp the arms toward the partition behind you.

Day 3: Daily Stretch Routine:

Follow the daily stretch routine as described above.

Day 4: Daily Stretch Routine + 3x Moon Salutations + Standing Poses + Standing Balances:

Daily stretch routine:

Follow the daily stretch routine as described above.

Moon Salutations:

The procedure for moon salutations has already been discussed above.

Standing poses:

The procedure for standing poses has already been discussed above.

Standing balances:

The important advantage of standing balances is that it strengthens the thighs (which have some practical uses).

Instructions:

1. From Mountain Pose – Tadasana bend the knees until the thighs are almost parallel to the floor

2. Keep the butt low

3. Bring the arms up towards the ceiling

4. Bring a slight back bend into the upper back

5. Hold 5-10 breaths

Day 5: Daily Stretch Routine:

Follow the daily stretch routine as described above.

Day 6: Daily Stretch Routine + 3x Moon Salutations + Standing Poses + Yoga for Abs:

Daily stretch routine:

Follow the daily stretch routine as described above.

Moon Salutations:

The procedure for moon salutations has already been discussed above.

Standing poses:

The procedure for standing poses has already been discussed above.

Yoga for Abs:

This categorization is made up of postures that will increase your core strength and help compress your abs. While doing yoga is not the finest way to get a six-pack, you can presume it will tone and make your stomach stronger. Solidification of your core can also help discharge back pain and mend your posture (nothing makes your belly look bigger than drooping!). Many of the postures recommended below are equilibriums, which are a great way to work the essential.

Let's get in full swing by coming onto all fours with your knees underneath your hips and your wrists underneath your shoulders. Do a few Cats-Cow Stretches to warm up, bending your back on your inhalations and rounding your spine on your exhalations. Remember to keep your belly tight throughout both motions.

Day 7: Daily Stretch Routine:

Follow the daily stretch routine as described above.

Chapter # 4: Week 4

Day 1: Daily Stretch Routine:

This has been described in the previous chapters.

Day 2: Daily Stretch Routine + 3x Surya Namaskara B + Standing Poses + Yoga for Arms + Seated Stretches:

Daily stretch routine:

Follow the daily stretch routine as described above.

Surya Namaskara:

The procedure for sun salutations has been given above.

Standing poses:

This has been described previously.

Yoga for Arms:

Tone your biceps and triceps for sturdy, sleek arms. Downward facing dog is done many times during most yoga classes. It is an intermediate pose, a quiescent pose, and a great strengthener in its own right. It may be the primary yoga pose you come across as you instigate a yoga practice.

Instructions:

1. Come to your hands and knees with the wrists beneath the shoulders and the knees underneath the hips.

2. Curl the toes under and thrust back raising the hips and straightening the legs.

3. Spread the fingers and push down from the forearms into the fingertips.

4. Stretch the upper arms extending the collarbones.

5. Let the head hang, then move the shoulder blades away from the ears towards the hips.

6. Employ the quadriceps powerfully to take the weight off the arms, creating a resting pose.

7. Pull the thighs inward, keep the tail high and sink your heels towards the floor.

8. Check that the distance between your hands and feet is correct by coming forward to a floorboard position. The space between the fingers and ends should be the same in these two postures. You should not step the ends/feet in the direction of the hands in Down Dog in demand the get the heels to the ground. This will occur ultimately as the strengths increase.

For Beginners: Try softening your knees, coming up onto the balls of your feet, bringing the belly to rest on the thighs and the sit bones up high.

Then sink your heels, uncurling the legs, keeping the high upward rotation of the sit bones. Also, attempt to move the arms somewhat out to the side, moving the torso towards the thighs. Then uncurl the arms.

Advanced: If you are very flexible, try not to let the rib cage go under the floor creating a dropping spine. Draw the spine in to maintain an even back. Try to hold the posture for about five minutes, retaining a block under your skull for sustenance.

Seated stretches:

The procedure has been given in the previous chapter.

Day 3: Daily Stretch Routine:

Follow the daily stretch routine as described above.

Day 4: Daily Stretch Routine + 3x Surya Namaskara B + Standing Poses + Standing Balances + Seated Stretches

These all factors have already been discussed before.

Day 5: Daily Stretch Routine:

Follow the daily stretch routine as described above.

Day 6: Daily Stretch Routine + 3x Surya Namaskara B + Standing Poses + Yoga for Abs+ Seated Stretches:

Daily stretch routine:

Follow the daily stretch routine as described above.

Sun Salutations:

The procedure for sun salutations has already been discussed above.

Standing poses:

This has been described previously.

Yoga for Abs:

This has been described in the previous chapters.

Seated stretches:

The procedure has been given in the previous chapter.

Day 7: Daily Stretch Routine:

Follow the daily stretch routine as described above.

Note:

You will require about 15 minutes to do your Daily Stretch Routine and 30-45 minutes to do your long-drawn-out routines.

Feel welcome to add more poses to your daily routine if you have time.

You can at all times take a yoga class as an alternative of your lengthier home practices if you desire.

Don't get disheartened if you skip a day of the planned schedule; rather just recommence your program the next day.

By finishing this 30-day introduction, you have come to be in the custom of doing a per diem yoga practice. Carry on practicing your short stretch routine daily and a longer practice three times a week and you will be well on your way to instituting a long-term yoga system that will recover your health and physical aptness.

Conclusion

The purpose of Yoga is to produce synchronization in the physical, vivacious, mental, psychosomatic, and spiritual aspects of the human being. In the preceding pages of this book, I have styled the Method of moderation in diverse postures such as stand-up, lying, and deskbound postures which carry synchronization. Yoga is not ordinary practice for an epoch or two in a day, but it is the most disciplined way of existing, all the twenty-four hours of the day. During the whole day, you may be solitary in one of these three postures and hence a skillful modification in them will affect the required synchronization. I have done my best to elaborate the essentials of yoga; now it's up to you to follow the book.

Good luck!

References

http://www.123rf.com/photo_31397649_young-woman-doing-yoga-exercises-outdoors.html

http://www.123rf.com/photo_20135033_woman-meditating-outdoors-sitting-in-a-yoga-position.html

http://www.123rf.com/photo_28865800_yoga-word-cut-out-of-white-with-clouds-and-sky-behind-it-along-with-benefits-of-the-meditating-exerc.html?term=yoga%20health%20benefits

http://www.123rf.com/photo_37061458_benefits-of-yoga.html?term=yoga%20health%20benefits

http://www.123rf.com/photo_30419233_schedule-of-the-day-woman-doing-sports.html?term=yoga%20schedule

http://www.123rf.com/photo_38931582_written-plan-yoga-class-on-calendar-page-background.html?term=yoga%20schedule

Author Bio

Muhammad Usman is a distinguished medical graduate of Allama Iqbal medical college (AIMC). He is a professional writer who has been in the field for more than 4 years. During this time he has produced 10,000+ articles, blogs and eBooks on various niches related to diseases, health, fitness, nutrition and well-being. He is a regular contributor to several journals related to medicine and surgery. He is the editor of several journals and newspapers.

Check out some of the other JD-Biz Publishing books

Gardening Series on Amazon

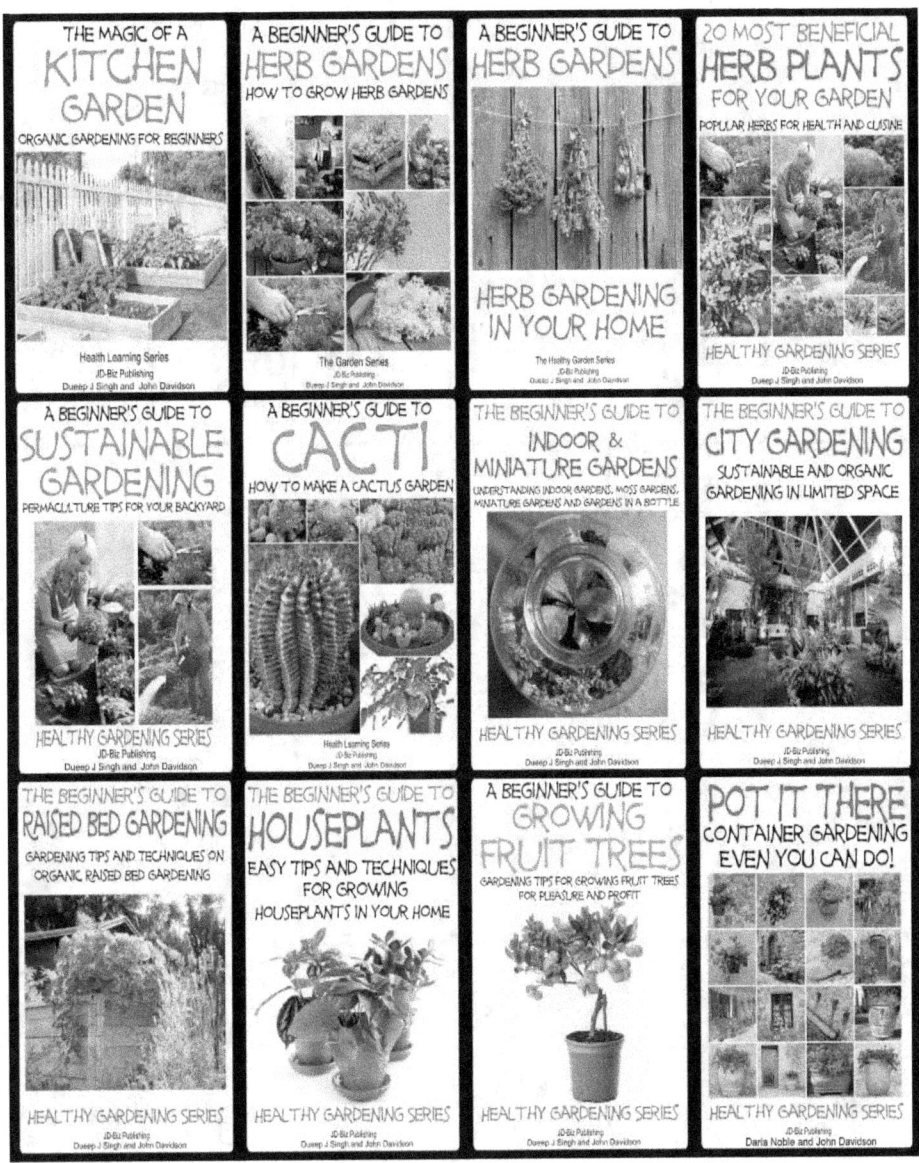

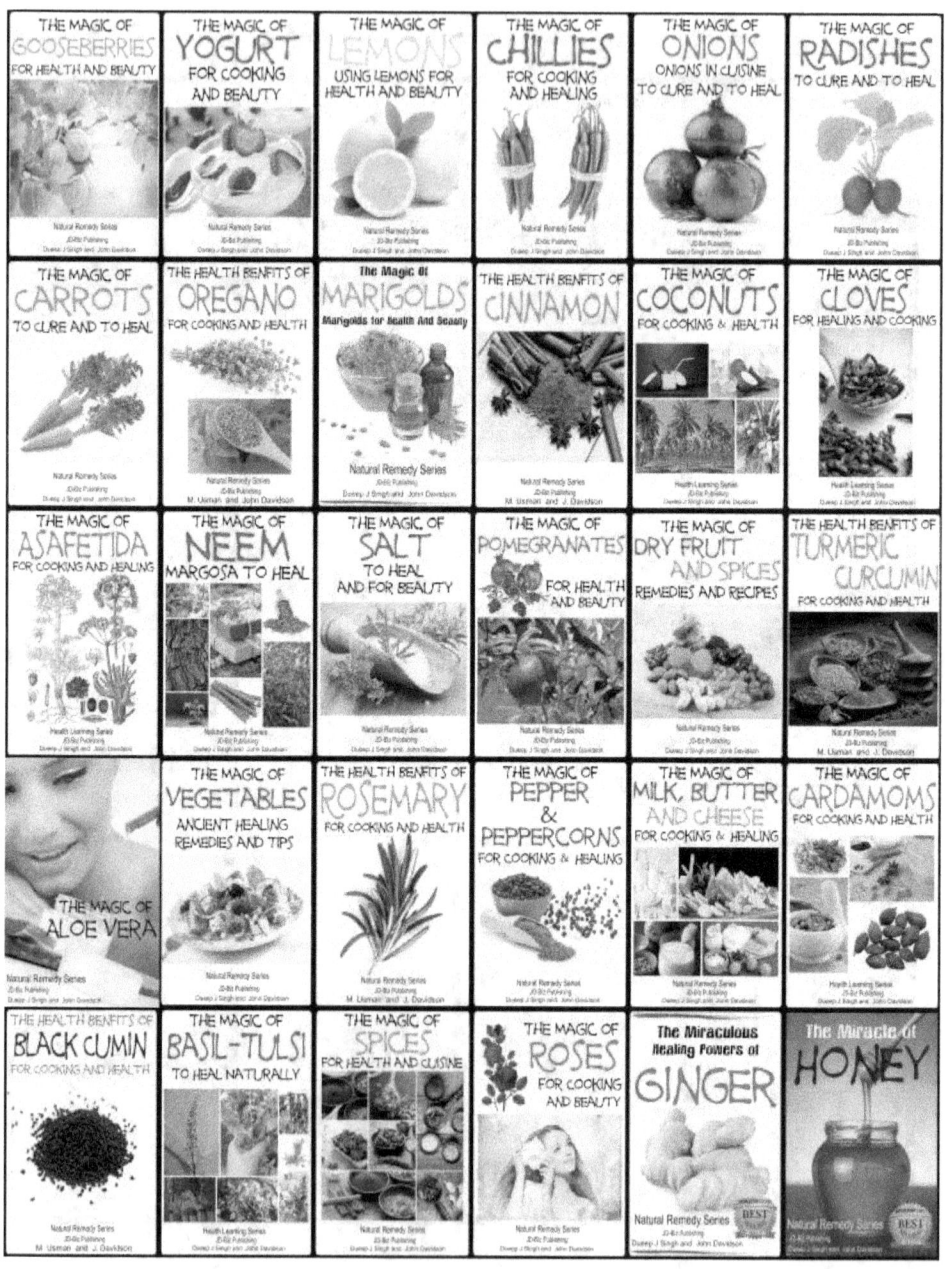

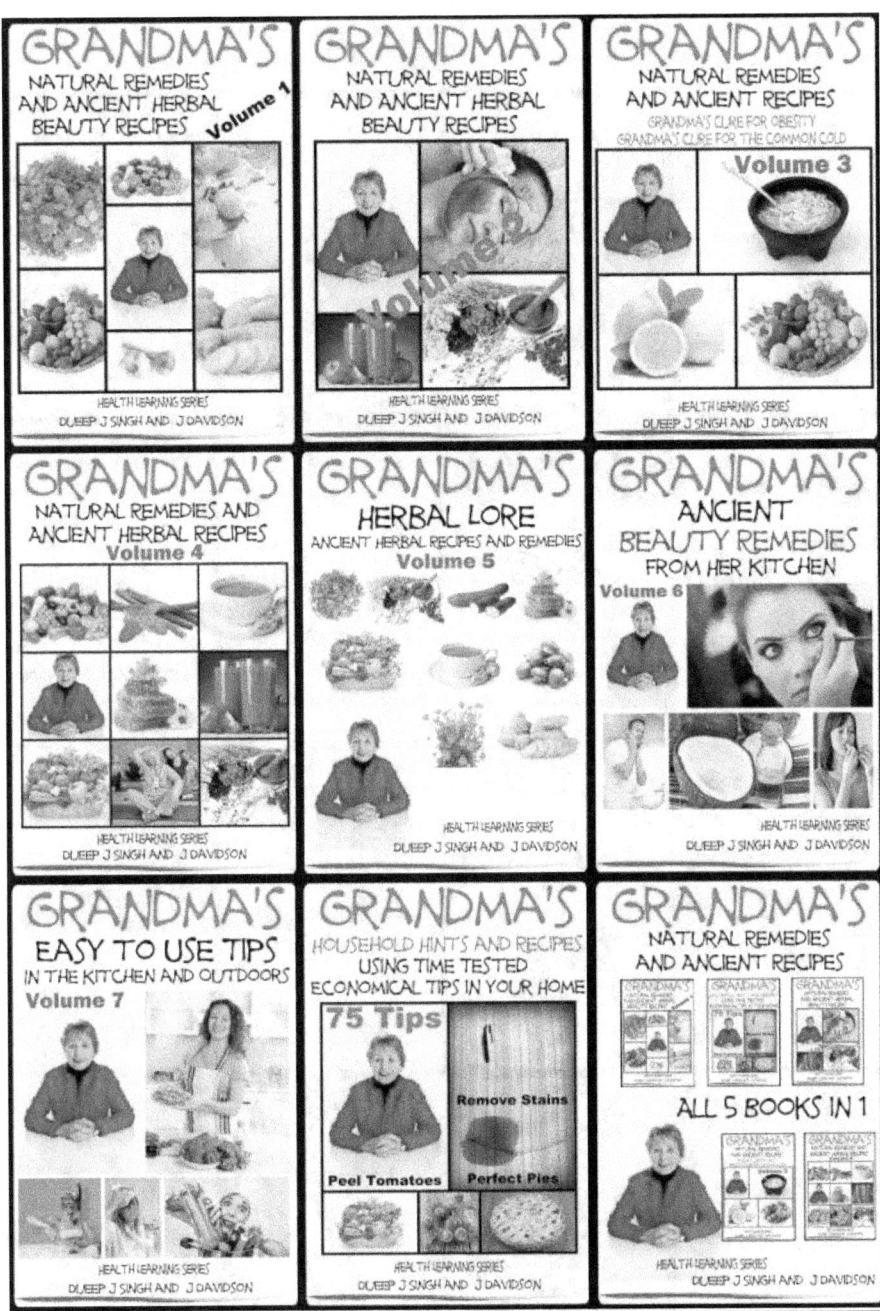

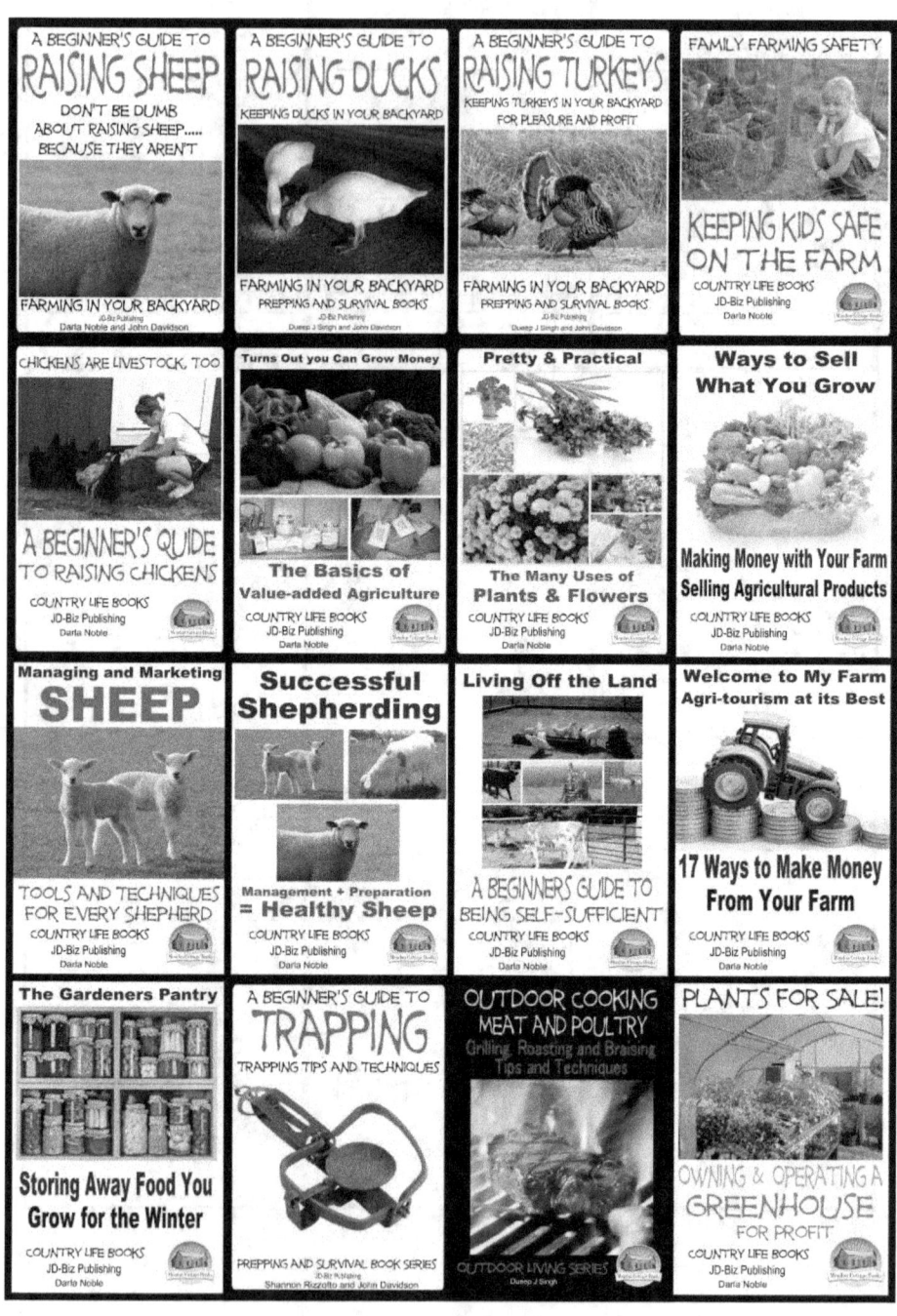

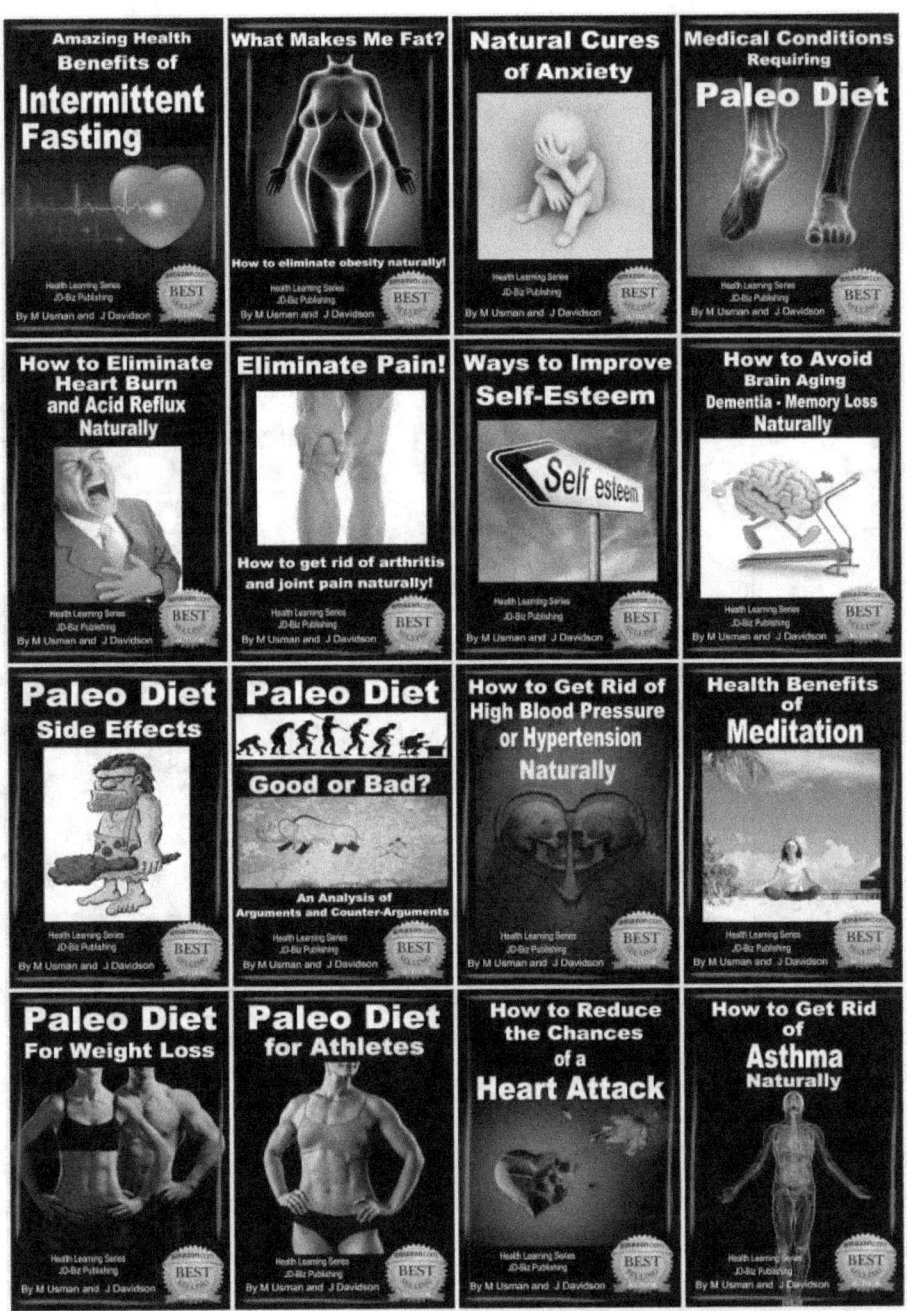

<u>Amazing Animal Book Series</u>

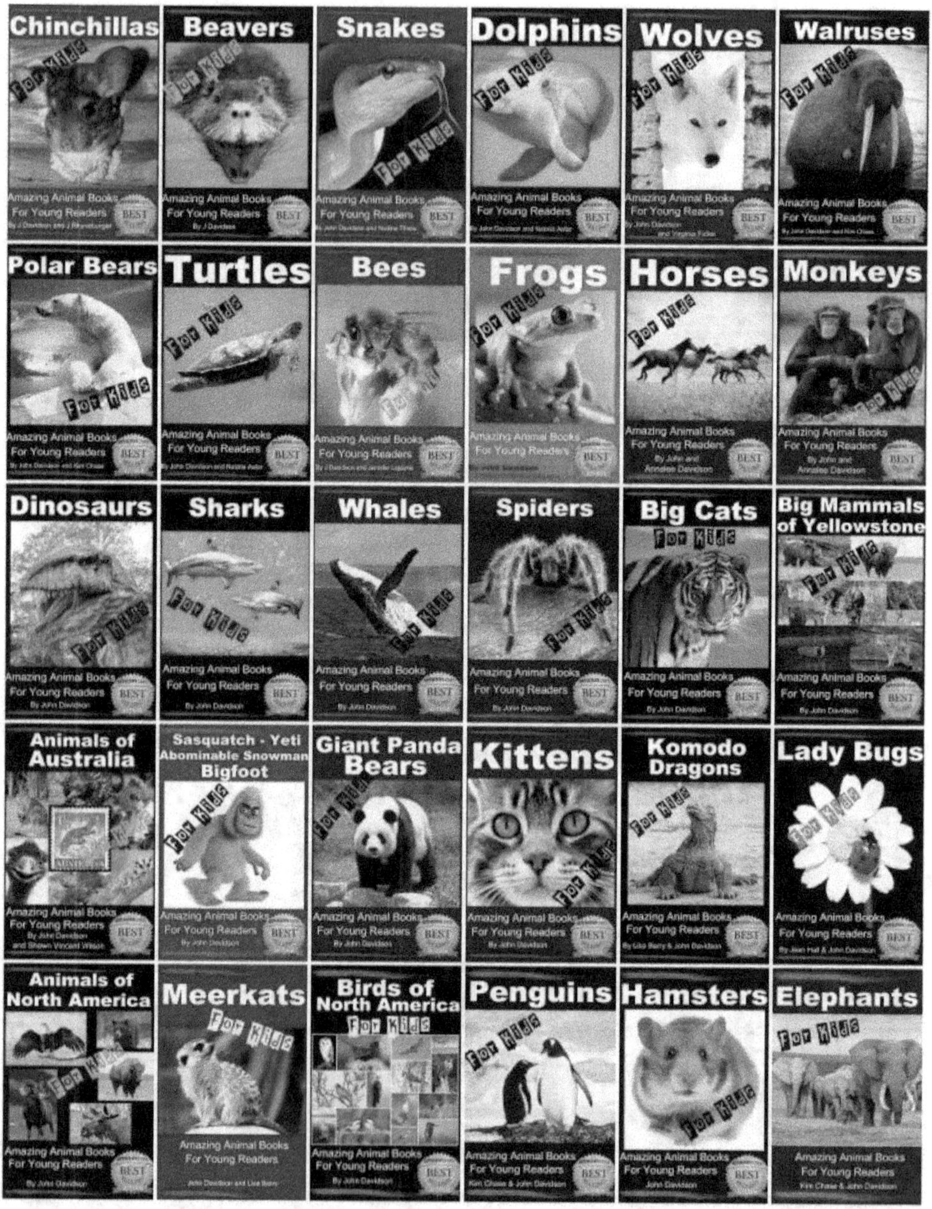

Learn To Draw Series

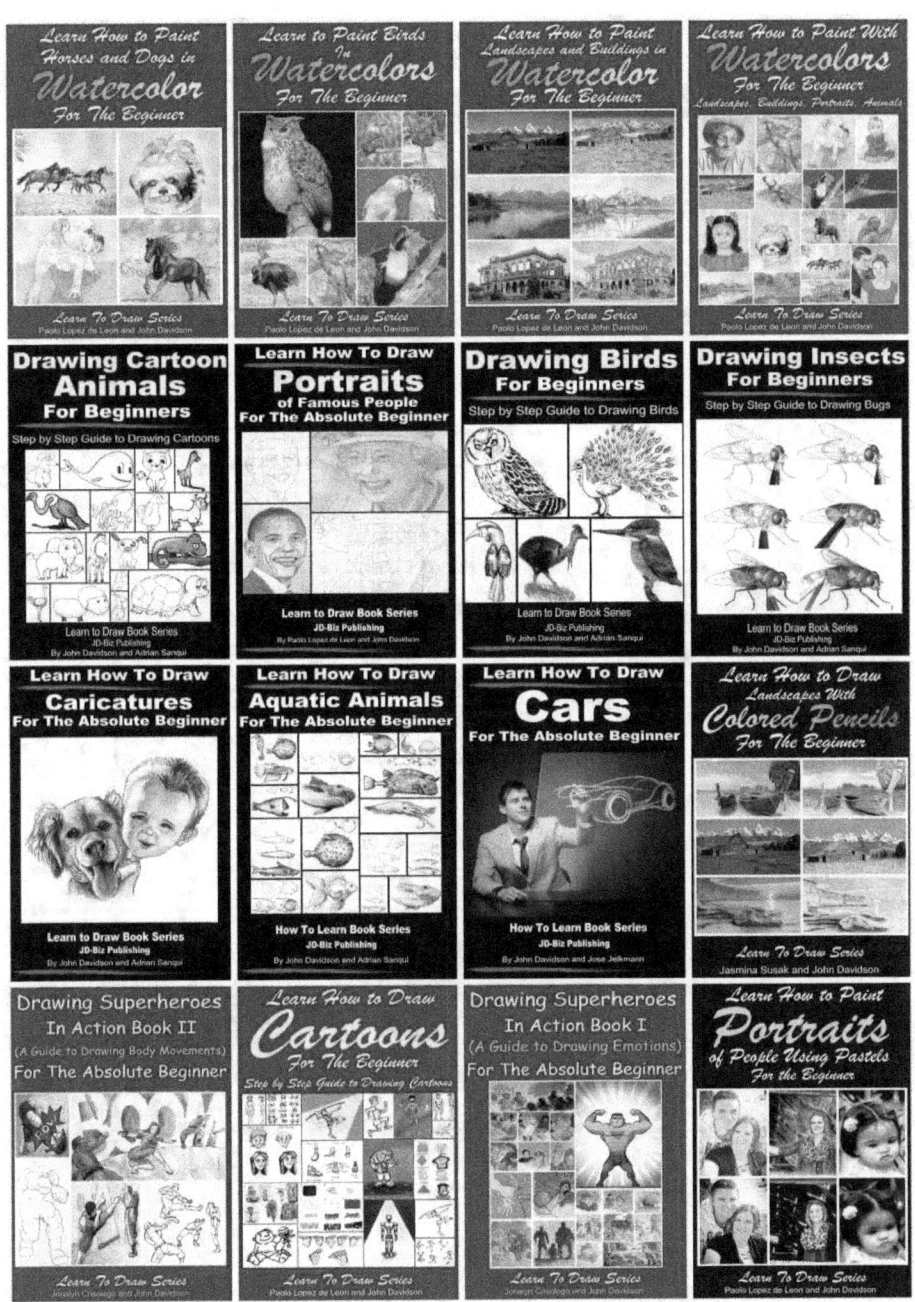

How to Build and Plan Books

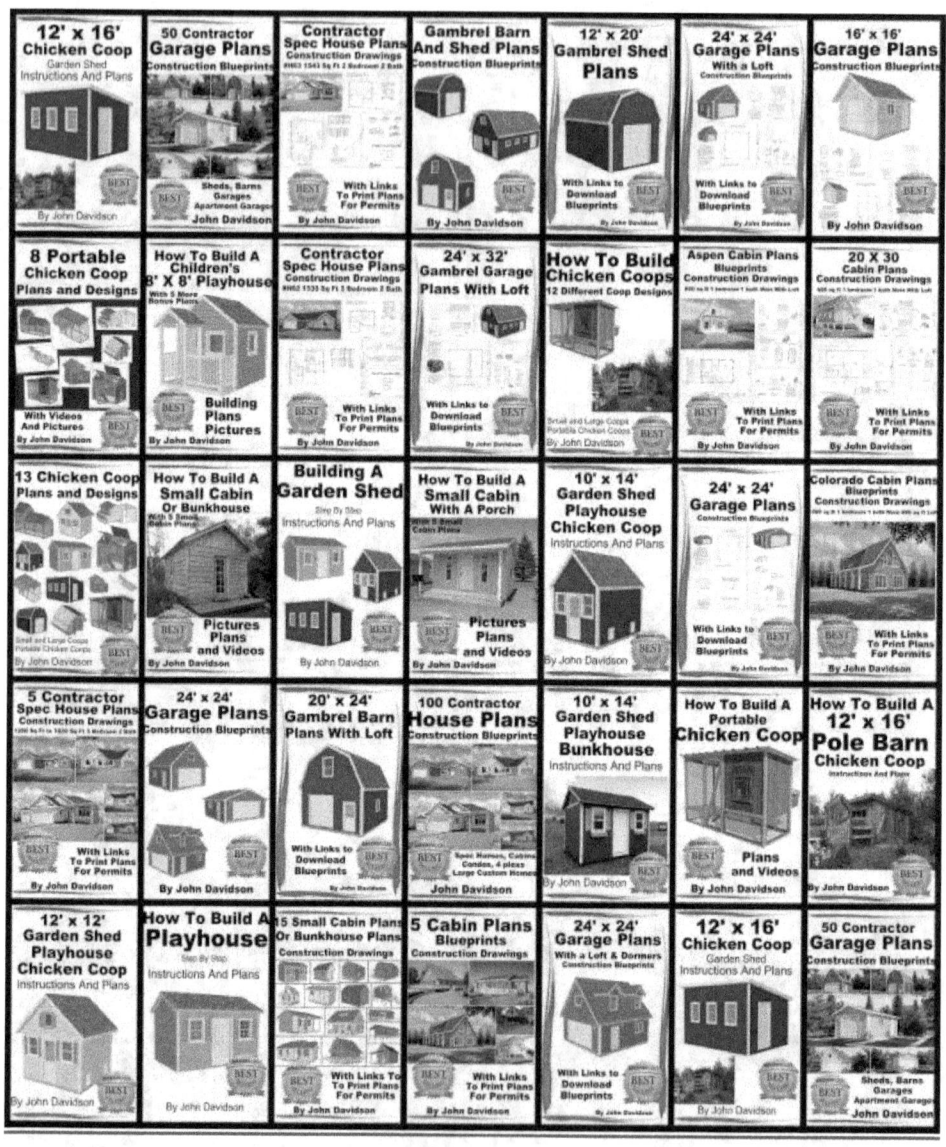

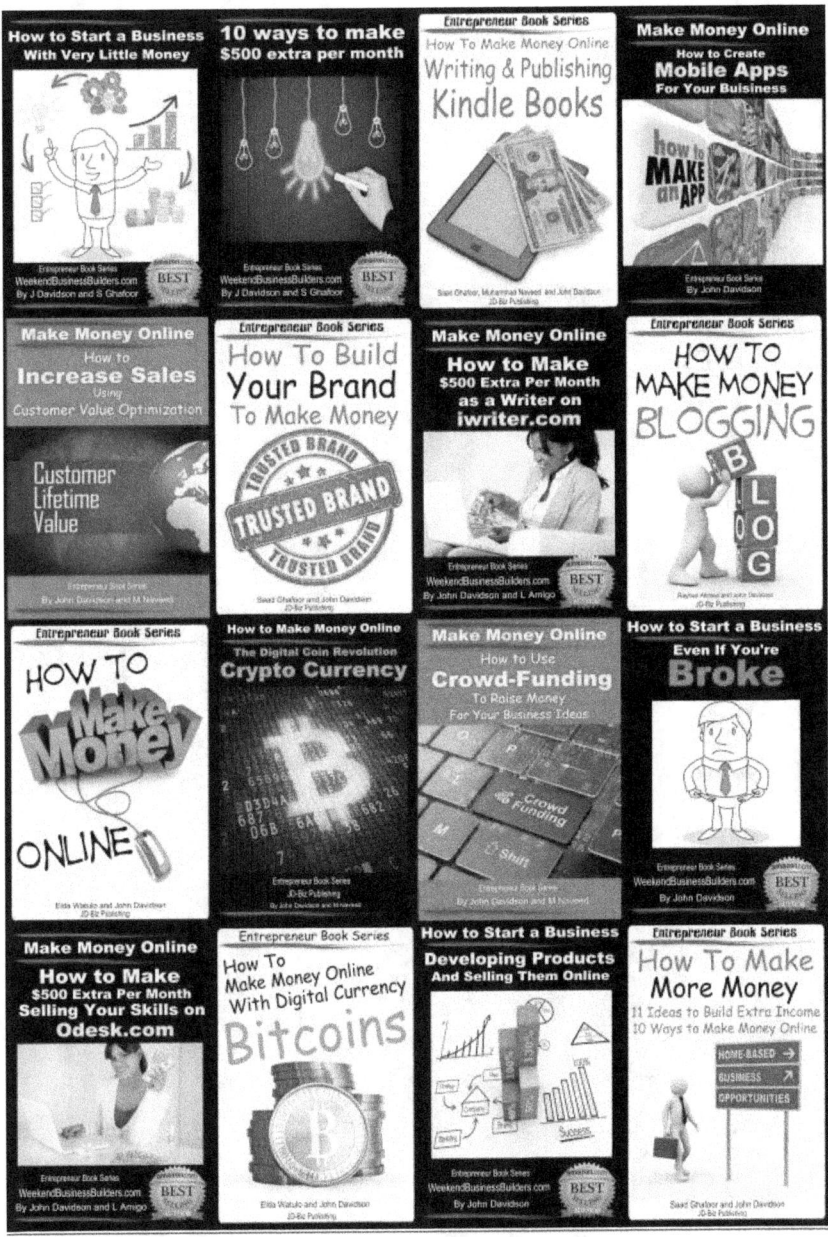

Our books are available at

1. Amazon.com

2. Barnes and Noble

3. Itunes

4. Kobo

5. Smashwords

6. Google Play Books

Publisher

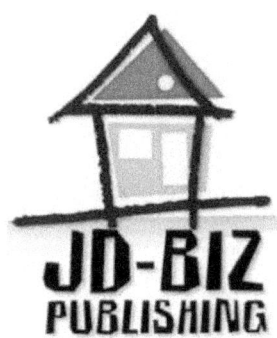

JD-Biz Corp

P O Box 374

Mendon, Utah 84325

http://www.jd-biz.com/

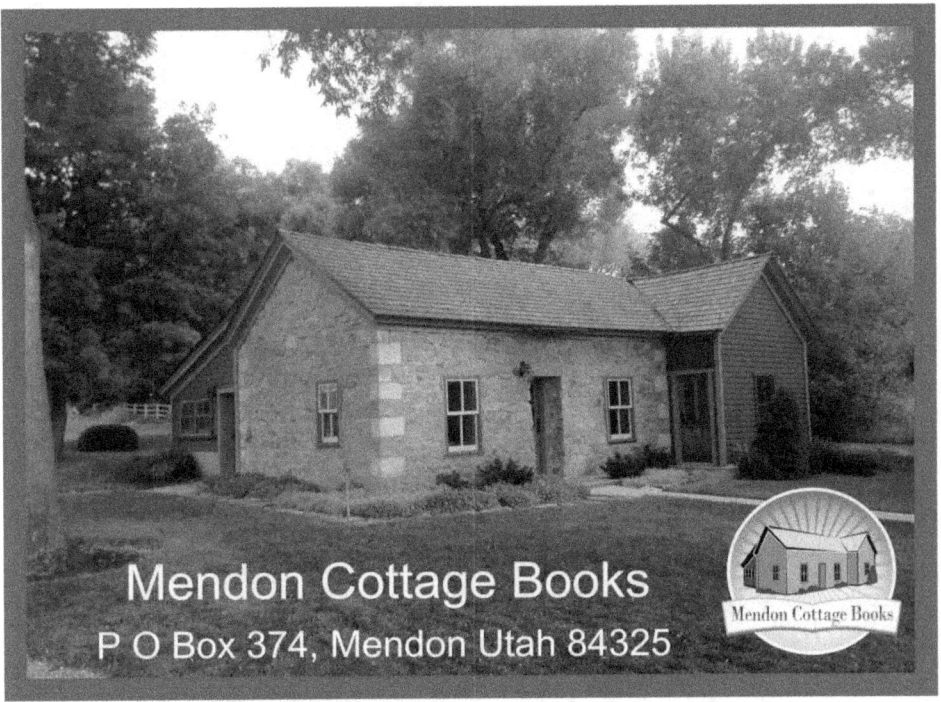